Keto Diet 101 - The Ultimate Keto Diet Book

Healthy and Delicious Recipes plus Simple Shopping Lists incl. 7-days Challenge

Elliot Black

ISBN - 9798835099191

Table of Contents

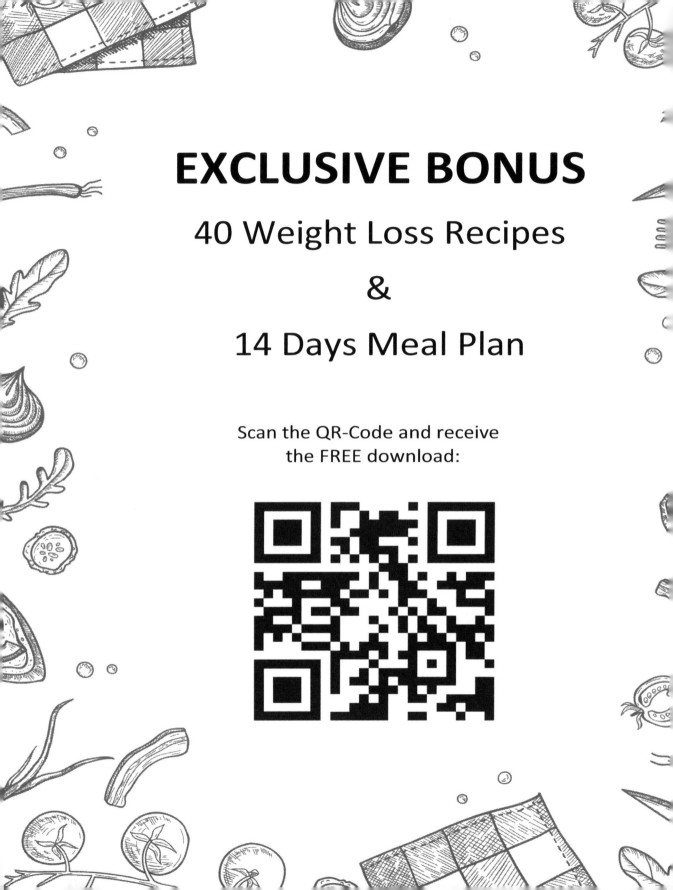

EXCLUSIVE BONUS

40 Weight Loss Recipes

&

14 Days Meal Plan

Scan the QR-Code and receive
the FREE download:

Introduction to the Ketogenic Diet

The ketogenic (keto) diet is a low-carbohydrate diet that has become increasingly popular in recent years.

There are three main macronutrients - carbohydrates, proteins, and fats. The keto diet involves consuming no more than 50 grams of carbs each day (usually those following keto aim for anywhere between 25 and 50 grams of carbs a day).

On this diet, you tend to consume a higher amount of fat and a moderate amount of protein. This will happen naturally because you are limiting your carb intake. The high-carb foods that were once in your diet are naturally replaced with high protein and high-fat alternatives. Usually, your macronutrient intake is split into 75% fats, 20% protein, and 5% carbs, but these percentages are slightly flexible.

The idea behind eating a low number of carbs on the keto diet is to encourage the body to switch to burning fats for energy. Usually, your body uses glucose for fuel. It breaks down glucose into something called ATP, which provides your cells with energy.

When you follow a keto diet, your body switches from using glucose to burning fats instead. These fats are broken down into compounds called ketones, which can be further broken down into ATP.

When your body enters this fat-burning state, it's known as ketosis. You will enter a state of ketosis after 3-4 days of following the ketogenic diet because your body will have used up all of its glucose energy stores by this point.

During ketosis, your liver starts to break down the fats that are stored in your body. It converts these fats into ketones that are used for energy when there is little to no glucose.

Being in ketosis has lots of amazing health benefits, which are discussed later in the book. One of the main benefits of the keto diet (and the most common reason why people switch over to a ketogenic diet) is its potential weight loss benefits.

It's important that, although you're on a low-carb diet, you should still eat a small amount of this macronutrient each day. Don't completely cut it out. You should still continue to eat some carbohydrates to ensure that you are still eating adequate amounts of plant-based fibre, vitamins, and minerals.

Eating a low carbohydrate diet might sound very restrictive. It's definitely not suitable for everybody but millions of people across the world follow a keto diet and absolutely love it.

This recipe book will make following the keto diet simple and easy. You can still enjoy all of your favourite meals, but you might need to adjust them slightly so that they are low in carbs. This way, you stay within your 50 gram a day carb limit.

This recipe book contains lots of recipes that cover all meals of the day, including breakfast, lunch, and dinner. There is also a seven-day meal plan at the end of the book to get you started on your new diet.

Every one of the recipes in this keto book is made using simple and easy-to-find ingredients. You can get all of the ingredients we have used in any UK, US, or Canadian food store. The recipes are perfect for beginners or advanced chefs, and they will be enjoyed by those who aren't following the keto diet too!

The nutritional values for every recipe have been included in this book. In particular, each recipe states the total number of calories, as well as the total number of carbs, proteins, and fats per serving. This should make things easier when you are calculating your carb intake each day.

The seven-day meal plan at the end of the book contains additional recipes to those that are listed in the breakfast, lunch, and dinner sections of the book so that you can switch things up and keep your keto meals interesting and varied.

Elliot Black

Who Should Follow the Ketogenic Diet?

Going on the ketogenic diet isn't appealing to everybody but it can be enjoyable. Millions of people choose to follow the keto diet out of choice but there are also many people across the world who follow the keto diet for health reasons.

Depending on your preferences and personal needs, the keto diet might be an ideal diet for you to follow. It's essential that you consult a professional doctor or dieting prior to switching over to the keto diet.

Drastically reducing your carbohydrate intake has the potential to cause side effects and adverse reactions if it's not done properly. A healthcare professional will be able to offer their expertise and guide you through the process to ensure everything goes smoothly for you.

Despite not being for everybody, the ketogenic diet is extremely popular, and it might be perfect for you. We have discussed the benefits of the keto diet in more detail below so that you can learn more about why millions of people choose to follow this particular low-carb diet.

There are certain groups of people who may benefit more from the ketogenic diet than others. In fact, low-carb diets are being used more and more in medicine as part of certain patients' treatment programs.

So, who should follow the ketogenic diet? In particular, the following groups of people will benefit from following the keto diet:

- People who are on a weight loss journey

- People who suffer from type 1 or type 2 diabetes

- People with hypertension (high blood pressure) or hypercholesterolaemia (high blood cholesterol levels)

- Those who enjoy eating a higher fat diet and aren't too bothered about eating lots of carbs

- People who are looking for a diet to boost their mental clarity and focus

- Alzheimer's patients may benefit from eating a low-carb diet

- Some cancer patients may benefit from this diet

Before we delve into the recipes of this book, let's take a look at the mini benefits of the ketogenic diet and the common mistakes people make when they are first starting out following this diet.

Elliot Black

What Are the Benefits of Low-Carb Diets?

Following the ketogenic diet can provide a range of physical and mental health benefits. Let's delve into these benefits in a little more detail.

The Keto Diet May Support Weight Loss

One of the main reasons why people begin the keto diet is to lose weight. When you reduce your carbs, your body is forced to switch to burning fats for energy. The keto diet is the perfect way to switch into a fat-burning state without needing to severely restrict your caloric intake.

Additionally, when you are forced to consume a lower number of carbs, you will naturally stop eating a lot of the refined carbs that are commonly found in the modern-day diet. This boosts your health and may contribute to weight loss.

The keto diet is higher in healthy fats than a standard diet. Fats are the most satiating macronutrient, so you will feel fuller for longer when you're following the keto diet. This makes it easier to reduce your caloric intake without feeling too hungry, so you can lose weight and reach your physique goals.

The Keto Diet May Reduce Risk of Certain Cancers

The keto diet can be used as part of cancer treatment and prevention.

Exciting research indicates that the keto diet may be beneficial as part of cancer treatment. Traditional cancer therapies work by increasing the oxidative stress inside cancer cells, which causes them to die. Studies have suggested that the keto diet may also have the same effects due to the low amount of carbohydrates in the diet.

Chronically high blood sugar levels are also linked to an increased risk of cancer. Since the keto diet is low in carbohydrates, it can help to lower blood sugar levels, and this can reduce the risk of cancer development.

The Keto Diet Can Lower Blood Sugar Levels

For people with type 1 or type 2 diabetes, following the keto diet can help to regulate blood sugar levels. In fact, the keto diet is recommended by medical professionals and dietitians to those who are suffering from diabetes because of its ability to decrease blood glucose, and therefore blood insulin, levels.

Eating fewer carbohydrates means that your blood sugar levels won't spike as highly or as often, and this directly reduces insulin spikes, helping those with diabetes to better regulate their insulin levels.

Studies show that the keto diet can reduce the required insulin dosage in those with type 1 diabetes by up to 50%.

The Keto Diet Can Improve Heart Health

Triglycerides are a type of cholesterol molecule that circulates through the body in the bloodstream. High levels of triglycerides in the blood can be a risk factor for heart disease. and their presence in large amounts can increase the risk of heart disease.

Low-density lipoproteins are known as the 'bad' cholesterol because they can increase plaque build-up in your arteries, which increases your risk of atherosclerosis and heart disease. High-density lipoproteins have the opposite effect and lower the risk of artery plaque formation.

Reducing your carb intake can decrease your blood pressure and your blood triglyceride levels. The keto diet decreases the levels of low-density lipoproteins and increases the levels of high-density lipoproteins. This can boost your heart health and lower your risk of heart disease.

The Keto Diet May Enhance Brain Function

Your brain usually uses glucose as an energy source but when you are on the keto diet and you're consuming a low amount of glucose, your brain switches to using ketones as an energy source.

There are several neurological disorders that cause cognitive decline. The severity of the symptoms of these disorders may be decreased with the keto diet. Studies have shown that those with Alzheimer's disease and Parkinson's disease experience a reduction in symptom severity after following the keto diet.

The keto diet has also been used as part of treatment for epilepsy, especially in children. It has been shown to reduce the severity and frequency of seizures. One study showed that 16% of children who were placed on a ketogenic diet became completely seizure-free after a short period of time on this low-carb diet.

Elliot Black

What Foods Can You Eat On the Keto Diet?

On the keto diet, there are certain foods that you should avoid to ensure that you stay within your 50 gram a day carb limit. But don't worry, there are plenty of that you *can* include in your diet when you're trying to stay low carb.

It's best to search for foods that are high in proteins and healthy fats, or those that are naturally low in carbs.

To help you get started on your keto diet, here is a breakdown of the types of foods that you can eat when you're following the keto diet:

- Red meats and poultry, such as chicken, turkey, beef (ideally, grass-fed), pork, and lamb

- Fatty fish and seafood, such as salmon, tuna, cod, haddock, white fish, prawns, shrimps

- Dairy products, including eggs, cheese, yoghurt, and cow's milk

- Meat-free protein alternatives, such as tofu and tempeh

- Dairy-free alternatives, such as dairy-free cheese and dairy-free yoghurt

- Plant-based milk products, including almond, cashew, hazelnut, coconut, oat, and rice milk

- Low-carb fruits, including oranges, berries, plums, pears, and peaches

- Low-carb vegetables, which includes most vegetables apart from starchy vegetables

- Nuts and seeds, which includes most types of nut, as well as pumpkin seeds, sunflower seeds, poppy seeds, and chia seeds

- Plant-based oils, particularly olive oil, sunflower oil, and coconut oil

Drinks that are ideal for the keto diet include water (still or sparkling), black coffee, keto coffee (also known as butter coffee), and black tea.

Of course, you can eat higher carb foods when you're on the keto diet but doing so makes it difficult for you to stay below your carb limit. Try to include as many of the above foods as possible so that you can enjoy a range of delicious meals while keeping your body in a state of ketosis.

Although these foods are 'allowed' on the ketogenic diet, it's important to remember that some of these foods can contain a high number of calories. If you're on a weight loss journey, limit your consumption of red meats, dairy, nuts, and oils if possible.

What Foods Should Be Avoided On the Keto Diet?

Now we've covered the things that you should aim to eat lots of on the keto diet, let's cover the things that you should avoid.

To put it simply, you should try to avoid foods that are high in carbohydrates so that you can keep your carb intake below 50 grams. Technically, you can still eat these foods but they're going to seriously limit the rest of your diet if you include lots of high-carb foods in your diet.

That's why it's recommended that you just avoid these foods altogether.

So, what foods should you stay away from when you're on the keto diet? Here are some of the key foods to stay away from.

- Refined grains, including wheat, barley, rye, pasta, noodles, bread, and cereal

- Simple sugars, including most ultra-processed snacks like sweetened chocolate, candy, ice cream, cookies, as well as pastries, honey, and syrup

- Starchy vegetables, mainly white potatoes, sweet potatoes, parsnips, turnips, and swede

- Low-fat products, including low-fat spreads and low-fat pre-packaged snacks

- Trans fats in the form of hydrogenated and partially hydrogenated oils

- Sauces, including ketchup, BBQ sauce, sweet chili sauce, ranch dressing, and more

- Sugary drinks, such as fruit juice, smoothies, sodas

Common Mistakes On the Keto Diet

The keto diet can be difficult to get your head around at first. There are some common mistakes that people make when they're just starting out.

Here are some of these common mistakes to be aware of so that you can avoid making them yourself.

Consuming Too Many Carbohydrates

The most common mistake that people make when they are following the ketogenic diet is going over their carb limit. Sticking to a carb intake of 50 grams or less each day is tricky, especially if you're used to eating many more than this.

It's easier to over-consume carbs when you're not properly tracking your intake, especially if you're eating lots of the high-carb foods that are listed above.

The standard Western diet contains a lot of carbs, so if you're switching directly from this diet into a keto diet, you might find it difficult at first. But over time, you'll find it much easier to stick to your 50-gram limit.

Giving Up Too Soon

A few days into the keto diet, you might feel like giving up. The first few days are always the worst because your body is getting used to burning fats instead of glucose. A lot of people give up during these first few days and go back to eating their normal diet.

It takes time to get used to eating a low-carb diet and it might be a few weeks before you start to see the positive health benefits of the diet. You need to be patient if you want to make significant progress. Don't give up and you will eventually start seeing progress!

Not Eating Enough Calories

When you cut out all of the refined carbs and simple sugars from your diet, you might naturally end up reducing your calorie intake. But it's important to try and replace these missing carbs with fat and protein sources so that you still reach your daily caloric needs.

Find lots of high-fat and high-protein foods to include in your diet. This will ensure that you are fuelling your body with great food while also remaining within your carbohydrate limit.

Eating a higher fat diet might seem quite intimidating at first, but your body needs this higher fat intake to replace the carbohydrates that you're lacking in your diet.

Recipes

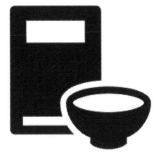

Elliot Black

Breakfast Recipes

Keto Chia Pudding

Makes 1 serving
Preparation time – 30 minutes
Cooking time – none
Nutritional values per serving – 276 kcals, 14 g carbs, 7 g protein, 20 g fat

Ingredients

- 3 tbsp stevia
- 2 tbsp cocoa powder
- 1 tsp vanilla extract
- 100 ml coconut milk
- 100 ml hazelnut milk
- 100 g / 3.5 oz chia seeds

Method

1. Mix the stevia and cocoa powder in a mason jar. Close the lid and shake well to ensure that there are no lumps.

2. Pour the coconut milk and hazelnut milk into the mason jar. Stir well using a spoon or close the lid and shake to mix.Add the chia seeds to the jar and either stir with a spoon or shake again.

3. Once the mixture has fully combined, place the mason jar in the fridge for 30 minutes to chill.

4. Serve with a sprinkle of extra stevia on top.

Elliot Black

Devilled Eggs

Makes 4 servings
Preparation time – 20 minutes
Cooking time – 15 minutes
Nutritional values per serving – 198 kcals, 5 g carbs, 16 g protein, 18 g fat

Ingredients

- 8 large eggs
- 4 tbsp mayonnaise
- 2 tsp Dijon mustard
- 1 tsp apple cider vinegar
- ½ tsp salt
- ½ tsp black pepper

Method

1. Bring a saucepan of water to a boil. Once boiling, reduce the heat to a simmer.

2. Add the eggs to the pan and cook for 12-15 minutes until hard boiled.

3. Turn the heat off, drain the water from the pan, and allow the eggs to cool.

4. When the eggs are cool enough and peel the shells off. Remove the yolks using a spoon, while trying to keep the egg whites whole. Place the egg whites aside while you make the sauce.

5. In a small mixing bowl, mix the mayonnaise, mustard, apple cider vinegar, salt, and pepper until fully combined.

6. Serve the eggs whites with some of the sauce mixture spooned in the hole of each one.

7. Serve with some low-carb vegetables or a side salad for breakfast.

Keto Peanut Butter Smoothie

Makes 1 serving
Preparation time – 5 minutes
Cooking time – none
Nutritional values per serving – 198 kcals, 4 g carbs, 6 g protein, 15 g fat

Ingredients

- 200 ml soya milk
- 2 tbsp smooth peanut butter
- 2 tbsp stevia
- 50 ml heavy cream
- 1 tbsp cocoa powder
- ½ tsp cinnamon

Method

1. Place all of the ingredients into a blender, except the cinnamon.
2. Blend until the ingredients form a smooth, consistent mixture.
3. Pour the smoothie into a glass and ½ tsp cinnamon on top.
4. Add some ice if you want to make the drink extra cold and enjoy.

Green Keto Smoothie

Makes 1 serving
Preparation time – 5 minutes
Cooking time – none
Nutritional values per serving – 132 kcals, 6 g carbs, 4 g protein, 10 g fat

Ingredients

- 200 ml oat milk
- 50 g / 1.8 oz fresh kale, chopped
- 1 celery stalk, chopped
- 2 tbsp fresh mint, chopped
- ½ avocado, peeled and sliced
- ½ cucumber, peeled and sliced

Method

1. Place all of the ingredients into a blender.

2. Blend until the ingredients form a smooth, consistent mixture.

3. Pour the smoothie into a glass.

4. Add some ice to make the drink extra cold and enjoy. If you prefer a fruitier smoothie, add some fresh strawberries and raspberries (note that this would change the calorie and macronutrient content of the smoothie).

Elliot Black

Keto Egg and Avocado Toast

Makes 2 servings
Preparation time – 10 minutes
Cooking time – 5 minutes
Nutritional values per serving – 310 kcals, 10 g carbs, 11 g protein, 14 g fat

Ingredients

- 1 tsp olive oil
- 1 large egg
- 1 avocado
- 2 slices keto bread
- ½ tsp black pepper

Method

1. Heat the olive oil in a small frying pan.

2. Crack the egg into the frying pan and cook for 3 minutes until the white of the egg is fully cooked.

3. While the egg is cooking, peel the avocado, remove the pit, and slice.

4. Toast the keto bread for a few minutes until lightly toasted and golden.

5. Add the avocado slices to one slice of toast and the fried egg onto the other slice. Top both slices with a pinch of black salt.

Keto Blueberry Pancakes

Makes 4 servings
Preparation time – 5 minutes
Cooking time – 10 minutes
Nutritional values per serving – 387 kcals, 9 g carbs, 12 g protein, 12 g fat

Ingredients

- 2 large eggs, beaten
- 50 g / 3.5 oz coconut flour
- 50 g / 3.5 oz almond flour
- 50 g / 2 oz cream cheese
- 1 tsp baking powder
- 50 g / 3.5 oz fresh blueberries
- 2 tsp vanilla extract

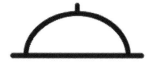

Method

1. Place all of the pancake ingredients in a bowl and whisk together until they form a smooth mixture.

2. Let the pancake batter sit for a few minutes and, in the meantime, heat a small, circular frying pan over a medium heat.

3. Pour one-quarter of the batter into the hot frying pan and allow it to spread across the bottom of the pan into a circle pancake shape.

4. Cook the pancake until bubbles begin to form in the batter. Flip the pancake over and cook for a further 2-3 minutes.

5. Once the batter is cooked on both sides and the pancake is a crispy golden colour, remove from the pan and set aside while you repeat these steps a further 3 times with the rest of the pancake batter.

6. Serve the pancakes topped with butter, heavy cream, or flavoured sugar-free syrup.

Almond and Peanut Butter Yoghurt Pots

Makes 1 serving
Preparation time – 10 minutes
Cooking time – none
Nutritional values per serving – 199 kcals, 19 g carbs, 21 g protein, 15 g fat

Ingredients

- 50 g / 3.5 oz strawberries, cut into quarters
- 2 tbsp almond butter
- 2 tbsp peanut butter
- 4 tbsp Greek yoghurt
- 30 g / 1 oz granola
- 30 g / 1 oz chopped mixed nuts (almonds, cashews, walnuts, or hazelnuts)
- 2 tsp chia seeds

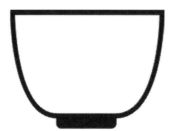

Elliot Black

Method

1. In a tall glass or narrow bowl, place half of the strawberries and add 1 tbsp each of almond butter and peanut butter.

2. Add 2 tbsp Greek yoghurt and all of the granola on top of the strawberries and peanut butter.

3. Place the remaining strawberries on top of the granola, followed by the final 2 tbsp Greek yoghurt.

4. Top with the second tbsp of almond butter and peanut butter and finish with the chopped mixed nuts and chia seeds.

5. Serve immediately while still cool and fresh.

Keto Cheese Bagels

Makes 4 servings
Preparation time – 15 minutes
Cooking time – 20 minutes
Nutritional values per serving – 220 kcals, 12 g carbs, 10 g protein, 25 g fat

Ingredients

- 200 g / 7 oz coconut flour
- 1 tbsp baking powder
- 100 g / 3.5 oz mozzarella cheese, grated
- 100 g / 3.5 oz cheddar cheese, grated
- 100 g / 3.5 oz cream cheese
- 100 ml almond milk
- 1 egg, beaten
- ½ tsp chia seeds
- ½ tsp black pepper
- 1 tbsp butter

Method

1. Preheat the oven to 200 °C / 400 °F and line a baking tray with parchment paper.

2. In a bowl, combine the coconut flour and baking powder.

3. Place the mozzarella and cheddar cheese in a heat proof bowl and heat in the microwave for 2 minutes in 30 second intervals until fully melted.

4. Stir the cream cheese into the melted mozzarella and cheddar and cook in the microwave for a further 30 seconds to heat through.

5. Transfer the melted cheese mixture into the flour before whisking in the egg. Mix until it forms a dough-like mixture.

6. Split the dough into 4 equal portions and roll each into balls. Gently press your finger into the centre of each ball to form bagels.

7. Place the bagels on the baking sheet and sprinkle the chia seeds and black pepper on top. You might need to press the seeds and pepper into the dough so that they don't fall off while the bagels are baking in the oven.

8. Bake in the oven for 15-20 minutes until the dough is cooked all the way through and the bagels are golden.

Veggie Omelette

Makes 2 servings
Preparation time – 10 minutes
Cooking time – 20 minutes
Nutritional values per serving – 213 kcals, 8 g carbs, 12 g protein, 15 g fat

Ingredients

- 1 tbsp olive oil
- 2 slices bacon
- 6 large eggs, beaten
- 200 ml milk
- ½ tsp salt
- 50 g / 1.8 oz cheddar cheese, grated
- ½ red bell pepper, sliced
- 50 g / 1.8 oz spinach, chopped
- 4 cherry tomatoes, halved

Method

1. Heat 1 tbsp olive oil in a small frying pan. Add the bacon slices and cook for 6-8 minutes, turning halfway through. The bacon should be browned and crispy.

2. Once cooked, remove the bacon from the pan and set aside on paper towels to drain.

3. In a bowl, whisk together the eggs, milk, and salt until fully combined.

4. Cut the bacon into small pieces and add to the egg mixture.

5. Pour half of the egg mixture into the frying pan. Cook for 5-7 minutes before sprinkling half of the cheddar cheese across one half of the egg mixture.

6. Add half each of the red pepper slices, spinach, and cherry tomatoes on top of the cheese.

7. Flip the 'non-cheese' side of the omelette over so that it covers the side with the cheese and vegetables.

8. Continue cooking for a further 2-3 minutes until the eggs are fully cooked.

9. Repeat steps 5-8 with the other half of the ingredients.

10. Enjoy the omelette while it's still hot.

Egg and Cheese Veggie Bowls

Makes 2 servings
Preparation time – 10 minutes
Cooking time – 20 minutes
Nutritional values per serving – 241 kcals, 15 g carbs, 15 g protein, 12 g fat

Ingredients

- 100 g / 3.5 oz baby new potato, halved
- ½ salt
- 1 tbsp olive oil
- 1 courgette, sliced
- 1 red pepper, sliced
- 1 onion, finely sliced
- 1 garlic clove, peeled and crushed
- 1 tbsp dried chives
- 4 eggs
- 50 g / 1.8 oz feta cheese, cubed

Method

1. Bring a saucepan of water to a boil and add the potatoes and ½ tsp salt. Cook for 10 minutes until they have begun to soften.

2. Heat the olive oil in a large frying pan and add the courgette, pepper, onion, and garlic. Cook for 8-10 minutes until the vegetables begin to soften and turn golden.

3. Make 4 holes in the pan and crack an egg into each one. Cooking for 5-7 minutes until the egg whites are fully cooked but the yolks are still soft.

4. Spoon of the egg and vegetable mixture evenly into 2 bowls and top with some feta cheese.

Keto Breakfast Casserole

Makes 4 servings
Preparation time – 15 minutes
Cooking time – 45 minutes
Nutritional values per serving – 489 kcals, 15 g carbs, 18 g protein, 21 g fat

Ingredients

- 1 large cauliflower, broken into florets
- 400 g / 14 oz cheddar cheese, grated
- 8 eggs
- 1 tsp salt
- 1 tsp black pepper
- 1 tsp smoked paprika
- 1 tsp chili powder
- 100 ml heavy cream
- 8 slices bacon

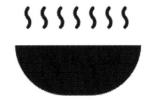

Elliot Black

Method

1. Preheat the oven to 180 °C / 350 °F and line a casserole dish with parchment paper.

2. Spread the cauliflower evenly across the bottom of the casserole dish.

3. Add half of the cheddar cheese on top.

4. Crack the eggs into a mixing bowl and add the salt, pepper, and chili powder, and heavy cream. Mix until combined.

5. For the egg mixture evenly over the cauliflower two coats the vegetables. Top with the remaining half of the cheddar cheese.

6. Add the bacon pieces on top and place the dish in the oven.

7. Bake for 45 minutes until set and crispy on top.

Elliot Black

Lunch Recipes

Keto-Friendly Mac and Cheese

Makes 2 servings
Preparation time – 15 minutes
Cooking time – 30 minutes
Nutritional values per serving – 411 kcals, 10 g carbs, 5 g protein, 18 g fat

Ingredients

- 1 large cauliflower, broken into florets
- 1 tbsp butter
- ½ onion, sliced
- 4 tbsp coconut flour
- 200 ml almond milk
- 2 tbsp heavy cream
- 100 g / 3.5 oz cheddar cheese, grated
- 1 tsp black pepper

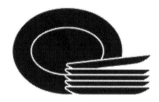

Elliot Black

Method

1. Preheat the oven to 200 °C / 400 °F and line a rectangular casserole dish with parchment paper. Place a large saucepan of water and bring it to a boil.

2. Add the cauliflower to the pan and cook for 8-10 minutes until softened. Drain and set aside while you prepare the cheese sauce.

3. Heat 1 tbsp butter in a large frying pan and cook the onion for 5-7 minutes until they become fragrant and start to turn slightly brown.

4. Stir in the coconut flour and reduce the heat to a low-medium heat. Cook for a further 3-4 minutes until the flour gets absorbed by the vegetables.

5. Pour in the milk and heavy cream. Turn the heat up to bring to a boil. Reduce to a simmer and continue cooking until most of the milk and cream have been reduced.

6. Remove from the heat and stir in the cheddar cheese and black pepper.

7. Add the cauliflower to the pan and mix well to coat every piece in the sauce.

8. Pour the cheesy cauliflower into the lined casserole dish and bake in the oven for 20 minutes until the cauliflower is hot all the way through and the cheese has melted. You can leave the casserole dish for a little longer if you prefer a crispier mac and cheese.

9. Serve while still hot.

Keto Zucchini Alfredo

Makes 4 servings
Preparation time – 10 minutes
Cooking time – 10 minutes
Nutritional values per serving – 279 kcals, 13 g carbs, 10 g protein, 13 g fat

Ingredients

- 2 tbsp olive oil
- 2 garlic cloves, peeled and minced
- 600 g / 21 oz zucchini noodles
- 100 g / 3.5 oz cream cheese
- 2 tbsp double cream
- 50 g / 1.8 oz cheddar cheese, grated
- ½ tsp salt
- ½ tsp black pepper

Method

1. Heat the olive oil in a large wok over a medium heat. Add the zucchini noodles and garlic and toss to coat in the oil.

2. Cook for 4-5 minutes until the garlic becomes fragrant and the noodles have softened.

3. Stir in the cream cheese and double cream. Cook for 1-2 minutes before reducing the heat to a low setting.

4. Add the cheddar cheese, salt, and pepper. Continue cooking for a further 3-4 minutes until the cheese has melted.

5. Serve while the noodles are still hot with an extra sprinkle of cheddar cheese on top.

Cheesy Garlic and Mushroom Chicken

Makes 4 servings
Preparation time – 10 minutes
Cooking time – 30 minutes
Nutritional values per serving – 356 kcals, 9 g carbs, 17 g protein, 16 g fat

Ingredients

- 2 tbsp olive oil
- 400 g / 14 oz skinless, boneless chicken breast fillets
- 1 tsp salt
- 1 tsp black pepper
- 200 g / 7 oz mushroom, sliced
- 4 garlic cloves, peeled and minced
- 200 ml heavy cream
- 100 g / 3.5 oz cheddar cheese, grated
- 1 tsp dried Italian herbs

Method

1. Heat 2 tbsp olive oil in a large frying pan and add the chicken breast fillets, salt, and black pepper. Cook for 10-12 minutes until the chicken has browned and is golden on top.

2. Remove the chicken from the pan and drain on paper towels. Leave the chicken juices in the pan.

3. Add the mushrooms and garlic cloves to the pan and cook for 5-7 minutes until the mushrooms have softened and begin to release water.

4. Reduce the heat and pour in the heavy cream. Simmer for 10 minutes, stirring occasionally.

5. Add the cheddar cheese to the pan and heat until it begins to melt.

6. Return the chicken to the pan and coat in the cheese mixture.

7. Serve with a delicious side of low-carb vegetables.

Carrot and Celery Soup

Makes 8 servings
Preparation time – 15 minutes
Cooking time – 40 minutes
Nutritional values per serving – 165 kcals, 12 g carbs, 4 g protein, 8 g fat

Ingredients

- 2 tbsp olive oil
- 3 carrots, peeled and chopped
- 4 stalks celery, sliced
- 1 garlic clove, peeled and finely chopped
- 4 vegetable stock cubes
- 100 ml milk
- 1 tsp salt
- 1 tsp black pepper

Method

1. Heat 2 tbsp olive oil in a large saucepan and add the carrots, celery, and garlic. Cook for 10 minutes, stirring frequently.

2. Meanwhile, bring 600-800 ml of water to a boil and dissolve the 4 vegetable stock cubes. Pour the hot stock into the saucepan along with the milk, salt, and black pepper.

3. Bring to a boil, then reduce the heat to a simmer. Cook the soup for 30 minutes until thickened.

4. Serve hot and store any leftovers in the fridge for a maximum of 5 days.

Bacon and Avocado Rolls

Makes 2 servings
Preparation time – 15 minutes
Cooking time – 5 minutes
Nutritional values per serving – 151 kcals, 5 g carbs, 10 g protein, 16 g fat

Ingredients

- 1 tbsp olive oil
- 4 slices bacon
- ½ cucumber
- 2 carrots,
- 1 avocado
- 100 g / 3.5 oz cream cheese

Method

1. Heat 1 tbsp olive oil in a skillet and add the bacon. Cook for 4-5 minutes until crispy and browned. Set the bacon aside to drain on paper towels.

2. Cut the cucumber, carrots, and avocado into thin slices, making them a similar size to the bacon strips.

3. Spread the bacon out on a chopping board or plate. Scoop some cream cheese onto each slice and spread it along the length of the bacon strips.

4. Add the cucumber, carrot, and avocado slices in layers on top of the cream cheese.

5. Take one end of the bacon strip and carefully roll it over to form tight bacon sushi-style rolls.

6. Serve hot or cold.

Steak and Aubergine Salad

Makes 2 servings
Preparation time – 10 minutes
Cooking time – 15 minutes
Nutritional values per serving – 312 kcals, 8 g carbs, 18 g protein, 14 g fat

Ingredients

- 3 tbsp olive oil
- 1 aubergine, thinly sliced
- 200 g / 7 oz sirloin steak
- 50 g / 1.8 oz feta cheese, cubed
- Handful lettuce
- 1 cucumber, sliced
- 8 cherry tomatoes, halved
- 2 tbsp vinaigrette

Method

1. Heat 1 tbsp olive oil in a frying pan and add the aubergine slices. Cook for 3-4 minutes, turning halfway through, until softened. Set aside to drain on paper towels.

2. Heat the remaining 2 tbsp olive oil in the same frying pan and add the sirloin steak. Cook for 3-5 minutes on either side.

3. Once the steak is fully cooked, set aside to drain on paper towels. When it is cool enough, cut into small chunks.

4. Create the salad by placing some feta, lettuce, cucumber, and cherry tomatoes into two bowls. Add the steak pieces and aubergine slices along with 1 tbsp of vinaigrette on top of the salad in each bowl.

Crispy Keto Taco Shells

Makes 4 servings
Preparation time – 10 minutes
Cooking time – 20 minutes
Nutritional values per serving – 354 kcals, 12 g carbs, 16 g protein, 15 g fat

Ingredients

For the tacos:

- 200 g / 7 oz mozzarella, grated
- 2 tbsp coconut flour
- 2 tsp psyllium husk powder

For the filling:

- 2 tbsp olive oil
- 400 g / 14 oz ground minced beef
- 1 tsp chili powder
- 1 tsp paprika
- ½ tsp salt
- ½ tsp black pepper
- ½ avocado, peeled and sliced
- 2 tbsp guacamole
- Handful lettuce, chopped
- ½ cucumber, sliced

Method

1. Preheat the oven to 175 °C / 350 °F and line a baking tray with parchment paper.

2. Add the mozzarella, coconut flour, and psyllium husk powder to a blender. Mix the ingredients until they resemble breadcrumbs.

3. Draw 4 circles of 15 cm / 6 inch onto the parchment paper and scoop the taco mixture onto each one.

4. Spread the mixture out so that it covers the inside of the circles. Press down each circle so that the top is even, and the edges are smooth.

5. Bake in the oven for 10 minutes until golden and crispy. As soon as they are removed from the oven, curve them over the side of a frying pan to form taco shapes. Allow to cool while you make the filling.

6. Make the filling by heating 2 tbsp olive oil in a frying pan and adding the ground minced beef.

7. Cook for 8-10 minutes, stirring frequently, until the beef is fully cooked and browned. Stir in 1 tsp chili powder, 1 tsp paprika, ½ tsp salt, and ½ tsp black pepper.

8. Reheat the taco shells by placing them in the microwave for 30 seconds.

9. Make the tacos by placing the taco shells on a plate and scooping some of the beef mixture into the centre of each.

10. Top each with avocado slices, guacamole, some chopped lettuce, and some cucumber slices.

11. Enjoy while the tacos are still hot.

Smoked Salmon with Bubble and Squeak

Makes 2 servings
Preparation time – 10 minutes
Cooking time – 20 minutes
Nutritional values per serving – 310 kcals, 15 g carbs, 17 g protein, 12 g fat

Ingredients

- 200 g / 7 oz new potatoes
- 1 tbsp olive oil
- 100 g / 3.5 oz white cabbage, finely chopped
- 1 onion, finely sliced
- 1 spring onion, finely sliced
- 1 tsp dried mixed herbs
- 1 tsp chives
- 2 x 100 g / 3.5 oz smoked salmon

Method

1. Preheat the oven to 200 °C / 400 °F and line a baking tray with parchment paper.

2. Place the salmon on the baking tray and cook for 12-15 minutes until the fish breaks apart with a fork.

3. Bring a pan of water to a boil and add the potatoes. Cook for 10 minutes until softened. Drain the potatoes and set aside.

4. Heat 1 tbsp olive oil in a frying pan and add the white cabbage, onion, and spring onion. Cook for 4-5 minutes.

5. Mash the potatoes and stir in the dried mixed herbs and chives.

6. Mix the white cabbage, onion, and spring onion into the potatoes and shape the mixture into small patties.

7. Cook the patties for 3-4 minutes on either side until golden and crispy.

8. Serve the salmon fillets alongside the bubble and squeak patties and a side of low-carb vegetables.

Keto Vegetable Soup

Makes 8 servings
Preparation time – 15 minutes
Cooking time – 40 minutes
Nutritional values per serving – 112 kcals, 5 g carbs, 3 g protein, 4 g fat

Ingredients

- 4 vegetable stock cubes
- 1 tbsp butter
- 1 tbsp olive oil
- 1 onion, peeled and chopped
- 4 garlic cloves, peeled and minced
- 2 stalks celery, chopped
- 3 carrots, peeled and chopped
- ½ large broccoli, broken into florets
- ½ large cauliflower, broken into florets
- 1 x 400 g / 14 oz chopped tomatoes
- 1 tbsp soy sauce
- 1 tbsp dried mixed herbs
- 1 tbsp dried chives
- 1 tsp salt
- 1 tsp black pepper
- 2 tbsp heavy cream

Elliot Black

Method

1. Dissolve 4 vegetable stock cubes in 600-800 ml boiling water.

2. Heat 1 tbsp butter and 1 tbsp olive oil in a large stockpot over a medium heat until hot.

3. Add the onion, garlic cloves, celery stalks, and carrots. Cook for 5-7 minutes, stirring frequently.

4. Add the broccoli and cauliflower and cook for 2 further minutes.

5. Stir in the hot vegetable stock, chopped tomatoes, soy sauce, dried mixed herbs, dried chives, salt, and pepper. Mix to combine.

6. Bring the soup to a boil before reducing to a simmer. Cook over a low to medium heat for 30 minutes. Stirring the heavy cream and continue to cook the soup for a few minutes until fully heated through.

7. Remove the stockpot from the heat and serve the soup while still hot.

8. Store any leftovers in the fridge for a maximum of 7 days.

Spinach and Mushroom Breakfast Casserole

Makes 4 servings
Preparation time – 15 minutes
Cooking time – 35 minutes
Nutritional values per serving – 231 kcals, 12 g carbs, 9 g protein, 16 g fat

Ingredients

- 1 tbsp olive oil
- 400 g / 14 oz mushrooms, sliced
- 400 g / 14 oz fresh spinach
- 4 garlic cloves, peeled and minced
- 1 tsp salt
- 1 tsp black pepper
- 1 onion, sliced
- 100 g / 3.5 oz cheddar cheese, grated
- 12 eggs
- 400 ml milk
- 1 tbsp dried chives

Method

1. Preheat the oven to 200 °C / 400 °F and line a rectangular casserole dish with parchment paper or grease with butter.

2. In a large frying pan, heat the olive oil over a high heat. Add the mushrooms and cook for 2-3 minutes.

3. Stir the spinach and garlic into the pan and cook for a further 2-3 minutes until the spinach has wilted. Sprinkle in the salt and black pepper.

4. Pour the mixture into the bottom of the lined casserole dish and spread out evenly. Add the onions and cheddar cheese evenly over the top.

5. In a large mixing bowl, whisk the eggs, milk, and chives together. Pour over the vegetables and cheese in the casserole dish. Crumble the remaining goat cheese over the eggs.

6. Bake for 30 minutes until the eggs are cooked and the casserole is golden on top.

Parmesan Chicken

Makes 4 servings
Preparation time – 10 minutes
Cooking time – 30 minutes
Nutritional values per serving – 319 kcals, 9 g carbs, 15 g protein, 17 g fat

Ingredients

- 2 tbsp olive oil
- 400 g / 14 oz skinless, boneless chicken breast fillets
- 1 tsp salt
- 1 tsp black pepper
- 200 g / 7 oz mushroom, sliced
- 1 onion, sliced
- 4 garlic cloves, peeled and minced
- 4 tbsp whipping cream
- 100 g / 3.5 oz Parmesan cheese
- 1 tbsp dried mixed herbs

Method

1. Heat 2 tbsp olive oil in a large frying pan and add the chicken fillets, salt, and black pepper. Cook for 10-12 minutes until golden.

2. Remove the chicken from the pan and leave to drain on paper towels. Leave the chicken juices in the pan.

3. Add the mushrooms, onion, and garlic to the pan and cook for 5-7 minutes until softened and fragrant.

4. Reduce the heat and stir in the whipping cream. Reduce the heat and simmer for 10 minutes, stirring frequently.

5. Add the Parmesan cheese to the pan and heat until it begins to melt.

6. Return the chicken to the pan and toss to coat in the cheese sauce mixture.

7. Serve while the ingredients are still hot with a side of low-carb vegetables.

Dinner Recipes

Beef Casserole

Makes 4 servings
Preparation time – 15 minutes
Cooking time – 1 hour 30 minutes
Nutritional values per serving – 245 kcals, 8 g carbs, 20 g protein, 13 g fat

Ingredients

- 400 g / 14 oz beef, diced
- 1 tsp salt
- 1 tsp black pepper
- 2 tbsp olive oil
- 200 g / 7 oz mushroom, sliced
- 1 onion, sliced
- 1 carrot, peeled and cut into small pieces
- 2 stalks celery, sliced
- 2 garlic cloves, peeled and minced
- 1 x 400 g / 14 oz can chopped tomatoes
- 1 tsp dried oregano
- 4 beef stock cubes, crumbled

Method

1. Season the beef with 1 tsp each of salt and pepper.

2. Heat the olive oil in a large saucepan and cook the beef 8-10 minute, stirring frequently, until cooked and golden. Add more oil or a bit of water if the beef gets too dry.

3. Add the mushrooms, onion, carrots, celery, and garlic to the pan. Cook for 5-7 minutes until the vegetables have begun to soften.

4. Stir in the chopped tomatoes, dried oregano, and crumbled stock cubes.

5. Add 600 ml of boiling water to the pan, bring to a boil before, then reduce the heat and simmer for 60 minutes.

6. Serve the stew while it's still piping hot.

Teriyaki Glazed Salmon

Makes 2 servings
Preparation time – 30 minutes
Cooking time – 15 minutes
Nutritional values per serving – 399 kcals, 7 g carbs, 21 g protein, 15 g fat

Ingredients

- 1 tsp stevia
- 2 tbsp soy sauce
- 2 tbsp avocado oil
- 1 tbsp rice wine vinegar
- 400 g / 14 oz salmon fillets
- 1 garlic clove, peeled and minced
- 1 onion, thinly sliced

Method

1. Preheat the oven to 200 °C / 400 °F and line a baking tray with parchment paper. Place the salmon fillets in the centre of the tray.

2. In a bowl, mix the stevia, soy sauce, avocado oil, and rice wine vinegar until combined.

3. Carefully pour the sauce evenly over the salmon fillets until they are all fully covered. Cover the fillets with tin foil and allow them to marinate for 20 minutes.

4. After 20 minutes, place the salmon fillets in the oven and bake for 12-15 minutes.

5. Remove from the oven and serve with a side salad.

Peanut Butter Chicken

Makes 4 servings
Preparation time – 15 minutes
Cooking time – 15 minutes
Nutritional values per serving – 245 kcals, 8 g carbs, 22 g protein, 14 g fat

Ingredients

- 400 g / 14 oz chicken breast fillets, cut into small chunks
- 2 tbsp smooth peanut butter
- 2 tbsp crunchy peanut butter
- 1 tbsp soy sauce
- 2 tsp brown sugar
- 2 tbsp hot sauce
- ½ tsp ground chili powder
- ½ black pepper
- 1 tbsp olive oil

Method

1. In a small heatproof bowl, combine the smooth peanut butter and crunchy peanut butter. Heat for 30-60 seconds until the peanut butter becomes more fluid.

2. Add the soy sauce, brown sugar, hot sauce, chili powder, and black pepper to the bowl and mix well.

3. Place the chunks of chicken in a large mixing bowl and pour the peanut sauce over the top. Toss to fully coat the chicken.

4. Heat 1 tbsp olive oil in a frying pan and add the coated chicken pieces. Cook for 12-15 minutes until the chicken is golden and crispy on the edges.

5. Serve the peanut butter chicken pieces with a side salad or some low-carb vegetables.

Chili Fish Salad Bowls

Makes 4 servings
Preparation time – 10 minutes
Cooking time – 20 minutes
Nutritional values per serving – 414 kcals, 17 g carbs, 21 g protein, 7 g fat

Ingredients

- 1 tbsp chili powder
- 1 tbsp paprika
- 1 tsp ground cumin
- 1 tsp cayenne pepper
- ½ tsp salt
- 1 tbsp olive oil
- 1 onion, sliced
- 1 garlic clove, peeled and minced
- 4 white fish fillets
- 1 red bell pepper, sliced
- Handful fresh spinach, chopped
- Handful lettuce, chopped
- 50 g / 1.8 oz sweet corn
- 1 carrot, peeled and thinly sliced

Method

1. Mix the chili powder, paprika, cumin, cayenne pepper, and salt in a small bowl.

2. Heat 1 tbsp olive oil in a large frying pan until hot. Add the onion and garlic and cook for 3-4 minutes until softened.

3. Sprinkle the spice mixture on the fish fillets and add them to the pan.

4. Cook for 12-15 minutes, flipping halfway through. You can test if the fish is cooked by using a fork. When cooked, the fish should easily flake and fall apart with a light touch of the fork.

5. Set the fish aside to drain on paper towels.

6. Add the red bell pepper to the pan. Cook for 3-5 minutes until softened. Add the spinach to the pan and cook for a further 2 minutes until the spinach begins to wilt.

7. Create the salad bowls by placing a bed of lettuce at the bottom of each bowl. Sprinkle some sweet corn and carrot slices on top of the lettuce.

8. Spoon some onion, garlic, pepper, and spinach into each bowl and top with the fish fillets.

Garlic and Soy Meatballs With Cauliflower Rice

Makes 4 servings
Preparation time – 15 minutes
Cooking time – 20 minutes
Nutritional values per serving – 356 kcals, 11 g carbs, 20 g protein, 15 g fat

Ingredients

- 2 chicken or vegetable stock cubes
- 1 large cauliflower, broken into florets
- 400 g / 14 oz ground minced beef
- 100 g / 7 oz cheddar cheese, grated
- 4 garlic cloves, peeled and minced
- 1 tsp oregano
- 2 tbsp olive oil
- 1 tbsp soy sauce
- Juice 1 lemon

Method

1. Boil around 600-800 ml of water and dissolve the chicken or vegetable stock cubes.

2. Add the cauliflower to a blender or food processor and pulse until the cauliflower forms a rice-like consistency.

3. Transfer the cauliflower rice to a large heat proof mixing bowl and pour the stock on top.

4. Cover the bowl with a microwave-safe plate and cook the cauliflower in the microwave for 5 minutes or until all of the water has been absorbed.

5. In a separate bowl, mix the ground minced beef, cheese, garlic cloves, and oregano until the beef is fully coated.

6. Use a spoon or your hands to scoop small chunks of the beef mixture to form meatballs.

7. Heat 2 tbsp olive oil in a large frying pan and add the meatballs. Cook the meatballs four at a time for 10-12 minutes each until brown and crispy all the way around.

8. When you remove the meatballs from the pan, set aside to drain on paper towels.

9. Pour the soy sauce and lemon juice into the bowl that contains the cauliflower rice and mix well to coat the vegetables.

10. Serve the beef meatballs on a bed of cauliflower rice and enjoy. Add a sprinkle of hot sauce for some extra flavour.

Stuffed Peppers with Chicken and Cheese

Makes 2 servings
Preparation time – 10 minutes
Cooking time – 50 minutes
Nutritional values per serving – 234 kcals, 17 g carbs, 16 g protein, 18 g fat

Ingredients

- 4 large red or yellow bell peppers, seeds removed and cut in half
- 1 tbsp olive oil
- 1 onion, sliced
- 2 garlic cloves, peeled and crushed
- 200 g / 7 oz chicken breast fillets, thinly sliced
- 1 tbsp Italian herbs
- 1 tsp salt
- 1 tsp black pepper
- 1 tbsp soy sauce
- 1 tsp lemon juice
- 100 g / 3.5 oz cheddar cheese, grated

Method

1. Preheat the oven to 200 °C / 400 °F and line a baking tray with parchment paper.

2. Place the pepper halves on the baking tray. Cook in the oven for 20-30 minutes until the edges are beginning to turn brown and crispy.

3. While the peppers are in the oven, heat 1 tbsp olive oil in a large frying pan over a medium heat. Add the onion slices and cook for 4-5 minutes until they start to soften and become fragrant. Add the crushed garlic and cook for a further 2-3 minutes.

4. Add the chicken breast slices to the pan along with the Italian herbs, salt, pepper, soy sauce, and lemon juice. Cook for 3-4 minutes, stirring occasionally.

5. Spoon the chicken mixture into each halved pepper and top with grated cheese.

6. Bake in the oven for 10 minutes until the cheese has melted.

7. Serve hot with a side of vegetables.

Beef, Mushroom, and Tomato Burger

Makes 4 servings
Preparation time – 15 minutes
Cooking time – 20 minutes
Nutritional values per serving – 468 kcals, 7 g carbs, 28 g protein, 21 g fat

Ingredients

- 400 g / 14 oz ground minced beef
- 1 tsp chili powder
- 1 tsp paprika
- 1 tsp BBQ seasoning
- 2 tbsp mayonnaise
- 2 tbsp olive oil
- 4 large mushrooms
- 2 large beef tomatoes, cut into 4 large slices
- 1 onion, sliced
- 30 g / 1 oz cheddar cheese, grated
- Handful lettuce

Method

1. Place the ground minced beef in a bowl and add the chili powder, paprika, BBQ seasoning, and mayonnaise. Mix to coat the beef in the spices and sauce.

2. Scoop the beef into 4 large patties.

3. Heat 1 tbsp olive oil in a large skillet and cook the mushrooms for 4-5 minutes before flipping over and cooking for 4-5 on the other side.

4. Remove the mushrooms from the pan and add the remaining 1 tbsp olive oil. Once the oil is hot, add the beef burgers and cook for 8-10 minutes, flipping halfway through. The burgers should be browned and fully cooked.

5. Remove the burgers from the pan and drain some of the juices. Add the 4 tomato slices and grill for 2-3 minutes.

6. To create the burgers, place the mushrooms on a plate and top each one with one beef burger, a few onion slices, and one tomato slice. Finish with some grated cheddar cheese and a handful of lettuce.

Chicken and Vegetable Stew

Makes 4 servings
Preparation time – 15 minutes
Cooking time – 1 hour 30 minutes
Nutritional values per serving – 211 kcals, 13 g carbs, 18 g protein, 8 g fat

Ingredients

- 2 tbsp olive oil
- 400 g / 14 oz skinless, boneless chicken, sliced
- 1 onion, sliced
- 1 garlic clove, peeled and finely sliced
- 200 g / 7 oz mushroom, sliced
- 2 carrots, peeled and cut into small pieces
- 2 stalks celery, sliced
- 100 g / 3.5 oz green beans, chopped
- 5 tbsp tomato paste
- 1 tsp dried mixed herbs
- 1 tsp salt
- 1 tsp black pepper
- 4 chicken stock cubes

Method

1. Heat the olive oil in a large saucepan and add the chicken. Cook for 7-8 minutes, stirring frequently, until the chicken has turned golden.

2. Remove the chicken from the pan and set aside.

3. Add the onion, garlic cloves, and mushroom to the pan. Cook for 5-7 minutes until all of the vegetables have softened.

4. Add the carrot, celery, green beans, tomato paste, dried mixed herbs, salt, and black pepper to the pan. Stir to combine the ingredients.

5. Place the cooked chicken into the pan.

6. Crumble the vegetable stock cubes into the pan and add 600-800 ml of boiling water.

7. Bring to a boil before reducing the heat down to low. Simmer the stew for 60 minutes until most of the stock has been absorbed.

8. Serve while hot and enjoy.

Coconut Fish Curry

Makes 4 servings
Preparation time – 5 minutes
Cooking time – 15 minutes
Nutritional values per serving – 342 kcals, 12 g carbs, 20 g protein, 21 g fat

Ingredients

- 400 g / 14 oz white fish fillets
- 1 tbsp olive oil
- 1 onion, peeled and sliced
- 1 garlic clove, peeled and crushed
- 1 tbsp garam masala
- 1 tsp chili powder
- 1 tsp turmeric
- 1 tsp salt
- 1 x 400 g / 14 oz can coconut milk
- 100g / 3.5 oz frozen peas

Method

1. Preheat the oven to 200 °C / 400 °F and line a baking tray with parchment paper.

2. Place the fish fillets in the centre of the tray and cook for 15 minutes until cooked.

3. Meanwhile, heat 1 tbsp olive oil in a large saucepan over a medium heat. Add the onion and garlic and cook for 4-5 minutes until the onions begin to become translucent and fragrant.

4. Sprinkle the garam masala, chili powder, turmeric, and salt over the vegetables and stir to coat. Cook for 1-2 more minutes.

5. Stir the coconut milk into the saucepan and bring to a simmer. Cook for 10 minutes until the coconut milk has thickened slightly.

6. Add the frozen peas to the pan and stir well.

7. Remove the fish from the oven and slice into small pieces. Add to the saucepan and stir to coat in the sauce.

8. Serve the curry while still hot.

Low-Carb Chicken and Vegetable Pizza

Makes 4 servings
Preparation time – 10 minutes
Cooking time – 15 minutes
Nutritional values per serving – 470 kcals, 17 g carbs, 21 g protein, 29 g fat

Ingredients

For the crust:

- 100 g / 3.5 oz mozzarella cheese, grated
- 3 tbsp cream cheese
- 100 g / 7 oz almond flour
- 100 g / 7 oz coconut flour
- 1 tsp salt
- 1 egg, beaten

For the toppings:

- 1 tsp olive oil
- 50 g / 1.8 oz chicken breast, sliced
- ½ onion, finely chopped
- ½ red pepper, finely chopped
- 3 tbsp tomato paste
- 1 tsp basil
- 50 g / 1.8 oz mozzarella cheese, grated

Method

1. Preheat the oven to 200 °C / 400 °F and line a pizza tray with parchment paper or grease it using butter or cooking spray.

2. Place the mozzarella and cream cheese in a saucepan over medium heat. Cook for a few minutes, stirring frequently, until the cheese has melted.

3. Fold the almond, coconut flour, and salt into the pan. Crack the egg into the pan and mix until fully combined.

4. Remove the dough from the pan and place it on a clean surface. Use a rolling pin to shape it into a large circle around 8-inch in diameter.

5. Transfer the pizza dough onto the lined or greased pizza tray. Bake in the oven for 10-12 minutes until the crust has turned golden.

6. While the dough is cooking in the oven, cook the pizza topping ingredients. Heat 1 tbsp oil in a frying pan and fry the chicken breast slices, onion, and red pepper for 5-7 minutes until fully cooked and crispy.

7. Remove the pizza from the oven. Using the back of a spoon, spread the tomato paste across the cooked pizza dough. Sprinkle the grated mozzarella cheese on top, followed by the chicken breast, onion, and pepper.

8. Return the pizza to the oven and cook for a further 10 minutes until the cheese on top has melted.

9. Serve hot with a side salad.

Tuna and Sweetcorn Mayo and Veggie Bowls

Makes 4 servings
Preparation time – 10 minutes
Cooking time – 10 minutes
Nutritional values per serving – 198 kcals, 6 g carbs, 15 g protein, 8 g fat

Ingredients

- 400 g / 14 oz canned tuna
- 4 tbsp sweetcorn
- 2 tbsp mayonnaise
- 1 tbsp Greek yogurt
- ½ tsp black pepper
- 2 tbsp olive oil
- 1 onion, finely sliced
- 1 red bell pepper, deseeded and finely sliced
- 100 g / 3.5 oz broccoli, chopped into small pieces
- 100 g / 3.5 oz carrots, thinly sliced

Method

1. Mix the tuna, sweetcorn, mayonnaise, Greek yoghurt, and black pepper in a bowl and set aside.

2. Heat the olive oil in a frying pan and add the onion, pepper, broccoli, and carrots. Cook for 5-7 minutes until the vegetables have softened.

3. Split the tuna and sweet corn mayo evenly into 4 separate bowls, followed by the cooked vegetables.

EXCLUSIVE BONUS

40 Weight Loss Recipes

&

14 Days Meal Plan

Scan the QR-Code and receive
the FREE download:

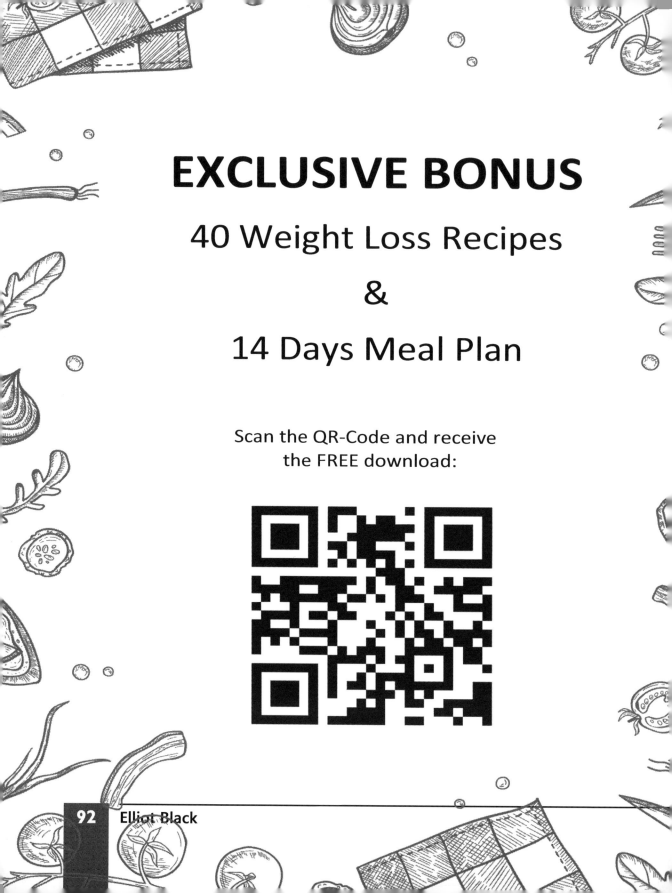

7-Day Keto Meal Plan

DAY 1

Breakfast - Sausage and Cheesy Eggs

Makes 2 servings
Preparation time – 10 minutes
Cooking time – 20 minutes
Nutritional values per serving – 303 kcals, 15 g carbs, 24 g protein, 20 g fat

Ingredients

- 4 Cumberland sausages
- 6 large eggs
- 2 tbsp heavy cream
- ½ tsp salt
- ½ tsp black pepper
- 1 tbsp olive oil
- 30 g / 1 oz cheddar cheese, grated

Method

1. Preheat the oven to 200 °C / 400 °F and line a baking tray with parchment paper. Cook the sausages for 20 minutes until fully cooked, turning them after 10 minutes.

2. While the sausages are cooking, crack the eggs into a mixing bowl and fold in the heavy cream, salt, and pepper. Mix until fully incorporated into a homogenous mixture.

3. Heat the olive oil in a large frying pan and add the egg mixture along with the grated cheese.

4. Cook for 5-7 minutes, stirring occasionally, until the eggs are cooked.

5. Remove the sausages from the oven and place two onto each plate. Add half of the egg mixture on top of the sausages.

Lunch - Bacon and Avocado Rolls (See page 54)

Dinner - Teriyaki Glazed Salmon (See page 72)

DAY 2

Breakfast - Almond and Peanut Butter Yoghurt Pots (See page 34)

Lunch - Avocado, Egg, and Tomato Salad

Makes 4 servings
Preparation time – 15 minutes
Cooking time – 15 minutes
Nutritional values per serving – 201 kcals, 8 g carbs, 16 g protein, 14 g fat

Ingredients

- 4 large eggs
- 4 tbsp mayonnaise
- 1 tsp lemon juice
- ½ tsp black pepper
- 2 avocados, peeled, sliced, and pits removed
- 4 beef tomatoes, sliced
- Handful lettuce
- ½ cucumber, sliced

Method

1. Heat a saucepan of water until it reaches boiling point. Decrease the heat down to a light simmer and add four eggs into the pan.

2. Turn the heat back up to boiling point and cook the eggs for 10-12 minutes until they are hard-boiled.

3. Remove the eggs from the pan and set aside to cool. Once cooled, peel the shells off the eggs and slice each one in half.

4. Place the egg halves in a mixing bowl and add the mayonnaise, lemon juice, and black pepper. Mix to coat the egg slices full in the sauce.

5. Plate two egg halves on each plate and prepare the salad.

6. To make the salad, add the avocado slices, tomato slices, lettuce, and cucumber slices to a bowl and toss to combine.

7. Serve the salad alongside the eggs and enjoy.

Dinner - Garlic and Soy Meatballs With Cauliflower Rice (See page 78)

DAY 3

Breakfast - Keto Cheese Bagels (See page 36)

Lunch - Smoked Salmon with Bubble
and Squeak (See page 60)

Dinner - Cabbage Stuffed with Beef and Vegetables

Makes 4 servings
Preparation time – 15 minutes
Cooking time – 1 hour 30 minutes
Nutritional values per serving – 346 kcals, 13 g carbs, 20 g protein, 15g fat

Ingredients

For the sauce:

- 1 x 400 g / 14 oz can chopped tomatoes
- 1 tbsp apple cider vinegar
- 1 tsp garlic powder
- 1 tsp onion powder
- 1 tsp dried mixed herbs
- ½ tsp black pepper
- ½ tsp salt
- 1 tbsp olive oil

For the cabbage stuffing:

- 12 large cabbage leaves
- 400 g / 14 oz beef, minced
- 400 g / 14 oz cauliflower, broken into florets
- ½ onion, peeled and sliced

Method

1. Preheat the oven to 200 °C / 400 °F.

2. Place the chopped tomatoes in a mixing bowl along with the apple cider vinegar, garlic powder, onion powder, dried mixed herbs, black pepper, and salt. Mix well.

3. Heat 1 tbsp olive oil in a large saucepan and add the tomato mixture. Simmer for 20 minutes until the tomatoes have reduced and become thicker.

4. To make the cabbage rolls, heat a large saucepan of water and bring to a boil. Add the cabbage leaves and cook for 2-3 minutes until slightly softened. Drain and set aside.

5. Add the cauliflower heads to a blender and pulse the cauliflower until it becomes a rice-like consistency.

6. In a bowl, add the beef, cauliflower rice, and onion slices. Mix well until it forms a consistent mixture.

7. Spread the beef and vegetable mixture across the bottom of a large casserole dish. Bake for 45 minutes until the beef is fully cooked.

8. Remove the casserole dish from the oven and use a spoon to scoop the mixture into the centre of each cabbage leaf.

9. Carefully roll the cabbage leaves up to form the stuffed cabbage rolls. Serve with a side salad and enjoy.

DAY 4

Breakfast - Cheese and Spinach Breakfast Muffins
Makes 4 servings
Preparation time – 5 minutes
Cooking time – 15 minutes
Nutritional values per serving – 101 kcals, 2 g carbs, 8 g protein, 10 g fat

Ingredients

- 8 large eggs
- 1 tsp salt
- 1 tsp black pepper
- 1 tsp garlic powder
- 100 g / 3.5 oz spinach, chopped
- 100 g / 3.5 oz cheese, grated

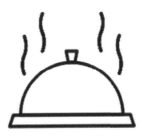

Method

1. Preheat the oven to 200 °C / 400 °F and line a 12-pan muffin tray with cases or olive oil.

2. Crack the eggs in a large mixing bowl and whisk together until combined. Add the salt, black pepper, and garlic powder.

3. Stir the spinach and cheese into the bowl and mix well.

4. Pour the mixture evenly into the 12 lined muffin cases and bake in the oven for 15 minutes until the eggs are cooked and set.

Lunch - Keto-Friendly Mac and Cheese (See page 46)

Dinner - Beef, Mushroom, and Tomato Burger (See page 82)

DAY 5

Breakfast - Keto Blueberry Pancakes (See page 32)

Lunch - Mushroom and Bacon Soup
Makes 8 servings
Preparation time – 10 minutes
Cooking time – 20 minutes
Nutritional values per serving – 308 kcals, 10 g carbs, 10 g protein, 20 g fat

Ingredients

- 1 tbsp olive oil
- 4 bacon slices
- 2 onions, peeled and sliced
- 2 garlic cloves, peeled and crushed
- 400 g / 14 oz mushrooms, finely sliced
- 4 chicken stock cubes
- 1 bay leaf
- 4 tbsp double cream

Method

1. Heat the olive oil in a skillet and add the bacon slices. Cook for 5-7 minutes until fully cooked, turning halfway through. Set aside to drain on paper towels before chopping into small slices.

2. In the same pan, add the onions and garlic, and cook for 8 minutes until softened and fragrant. Add the mushrooms and cook on a high heat for a further 3-4 minutes, stirring occasionally.

3. Transfer the bacon, onions, garlic, and mushrooms into a large saucepan. Crumble in the chicken stock cubes and add the bay leaf.

4. Simmer the mixture for 10 minutes before removing the bay leaf.

5. Transfer the mixture into a blender and pulse until it creates a smooth consistency.

6. Reheat the soup in a saucepan and stir in the double cream. Stir until the mixture is hot and serve.

7. Store any leftover soup in the fridge for a maximum of 5 days.

Dinner - Low-Carb Chicken and Vegetable Pizza (See page 88)

DAY 6

Breakfast - Keto Egg and Avocado Toast (See page 31)

Lunch - Cheesy Garlic and Mushroom
Chicken (See page 50)

Dinner - Cauliflower with Tomato and Cashew Sauce
Makes 4 servings
Preparation time – 10 minutes
Cooking time – 45 minutes
Nutritional values per serving – 267 kcals, 11 g carbs, 6 g protein, 10 g fat

Ingredients

- 1 cauliflower, broken into florets
- 2 tbsp cashews
- 2 tsp pumpkin seeds
- 2 tbsp vegetable oil
- 3 tsp garam masala
- 2 garlic cloves, peeled crushed
- 1 x 400 g / 14 oz can chopped tomatoes
- 2 tbsp cashew butter
- 2 tbsp double cream

Method

1. Preheat the oven to 200 °C / 400 °F.

2. Spread the cauliflower florets, cashews, and pumpkin seeds onto a baking tray. Spread 1 tbsp olive oil and 3 tsp garam masala over the top of the ingredients so that they are all evenly coated. Bake in the oven for 40 minutes until the cauliflower is soft and crispy on the edges.

3. Meanwhile, heat the remaining 1 tbsp olive oil in a large skillet and fry the garlic for 5 minutes. Add the chopped tomatoes and simmer for 15 minutes until they begin to thicken.

4. Stir in the cashew butter and double cream.

5. Remove the cauliflower from the oven and serve topped with the tomato and cashew sauce.

Elliot Black

DAY 7

Breakfast - Keto Oatmeal
Makes 1 serving
Preparation time – 5 minutes
Cooking time – 10 minutes
Nutritional values per serving – 355 kcals, 20 g carbs, 10 g protein, 10 g fat

Ingredients

- 2 tbsp flaxseed
- 2 tbsp almond flour
- 2 tbsp coconut flour
- 2 tbsp chia seeds
- 2 tbsp heavy cream
- 1 tsp vanilla extract
- 1 tbsp peanut butter
- 1 tsp sugar-free syrup

Method

1. Mix the flaxseed, almond flour, coconut flour, and chia seeds in a bowl. Stir to combine.

2. Add the heavy cream, vanilla extract, and peanut butter to the bowl and mix well.

3. Transfer the mixture to a saucepan and cook over a medium heat for 10 minutes until the dry ingredients have absorbed most of the wet ingredients. Add more water if the mixture is too dry.

4. Pour into a bowl and enjoy with some sugar-free syrup and a sprinkle of cinnamon or cocoa powder.

Lunch - Keto Vegetable Soup (See page 62)

Dinner - Peanut Butter Chicken (See page 74)

EXCLUSIVE BONUS

40 Weight Loss Recipes

&

14 Days Meal Plan

Scan the QR-Code and receive
the FREE download:

Disclaimer

This book contains opinions and ideas of the author and is meant to teach the reader informative and helpful knowledge while due care should be taken by the user in the application of the information provided. The instructions and strategies are possibly not right for every reader and there is no guarantee that they work for everyone. Using this book and implementing the information/recipes therein contained is explicitly your own responsibility and risk. This work with all its contents, does not guarantee correctness, completion, quality or correctness of the provided information. Misinformation or misprints cannot be completely eliminated.

Printed in Great Britain
by Amazon